Students Instruction Manual

Standard Peking Tai Chi Chuan Form

By

Master Richard Kosch

Students Instruction Manual
Standard Peking Tai Chi Chuan Form

By

Master Richard Kosch

Copyright 2012

Email: Sifurichkosch@yahoo.com

www.about.me/sifurichkosch

or take a snap with your smart phone to go directly to the web page

I first met Richard Kosch shortly after he had returned home from the Persian Gulf. He was in the Tai Chi class, and I was in the Northern Shao Lin Class. Two opposite sides of the Kung Fu scale. I had learned Tai Chi earlier but went on to Shao Lin, and most of the time our paths didn't cross, except on Friday nights when we'd all gather with our instructor to learn Chi Gong practice such as Yi Jin Jing, Ba Dua Jin and the ubiquitous Universal Post standing Chi Gong Meditation. We'd all be standing in Universal Post, which was not easy, but was made much more amenable by hearing old tales of China and the old Chinese legends of bygone masters.

Occasionally, Richard and I would meet up on sparring nights and at tournaments where I'd be competing in Shao Lin, and he, in Tai Chi. That was back in the mid-nineties.

Richard went on to teach Tai Chi, and I, to teaching my own brand of Shao Lin. We also went on to judge at tournaments. Later, he was very instrumental in helping to keep me in check when I was asked to develop a therapeutic Tai Chi system for health care, and today, we still continue to train on common ground, and to bring our form of excellence to tournaments where we try to encourage competitors. Did I mention that Richard was honored with Man of the Year for Tai Chi Instruction, 2006 from the World Karate Union? He has been recognized by several organizations for his continued contribution to Tai Chi, including his course: Tai Chi Principles for Massage Therapy.

I'm very proud to say that I have had the pleasure to train along side of Richard over these almost twenty years and to be involved with this project. I am also very proud to call him my brother.

Master Khadi Madama, Founder of Fa Shen Chuan Fa

February 4, 2012

It is my great pleasure to attest to the character and internal martial arts proficiency of Master Richard Kosch, on the occasion of the completion of his first book. As of this writing, I have been a training brother and student of Master Rich for over 15 years. He is an exemplary individual, having the utmost dedication to the arts he loves, evidenced not only by the distinctively high level of skill he has attained therein, but just as (if not more) importantly, the highest level of moral integrity with which he practices and teaches them. Master Rich brings great honor to the martial arts and continues to do so with this authoritative and trustworthy work.

Respectfully in the Martial Arts,

Master Brandon Underwood

February 2012

BIO OF SIFU RICH

Richard Kosch began studying Tai Chi Chuan in 1995 and by 1999 he was already a Black Belt recognized with the title of Sifu. This began his teaching career as well as his involvement in helping to develop an effective Tai Chi Program for Massage Therapy.

Richard has competed and won awards in Push Hands Competitions, demonstrated Tai Chi Chuan at various civic organizations and has remained active in the pursuit of excellence in his own practice.

His awards are numerous and he can trace his Martial Arts lineage back to the legendary Kuo of Chinatown, San Francisco and beyond that to China, where he is registered with the Chinese Historical Society, and the Traditional Chinese Medicine and Chi Gong Federation.

GETTING READY TO PERFORM THE
PEKING STANDARD YANG STYLE SHORT FORM

ORIENTING YOURSELF FOR PRACTICING THE FORM:

The Peking Form utilized the four compass points of;
North
South
East
West.

These directions are oriented to where you are facing, not necessarily the actual magnetic compass points. In other words, wherever you are facing is considered North, and so forth.

GLOSSARY

Tan Tien: refers to the area just below the naval. The Chinese consider this to be a powerful energy center. It is also your physical center of gravity.

A NOTE FROM SIFU RICH:

Spend 10 minutes of staying in the space of the form focusing within. An old story illustrates this practice.

One day the old Chinese master was sitting in the garden having tea with his student. The student tells the master that he wants to be the greatest master in the world and asks the master what is the secret to being the greatest. The old master replied " You can learn the secret by listening to the flower". The student pondered this for awhile and went off to try to learn the secret of the flower. He returned to the master and told him "Master, I have heard nothing". "Exactly", the master replied.

TAI CHI CHUAN STANDARD

WARM UPS

Tai Chi Chuan Standard Warm Up Movements

1. Ankle Rotations
2. Knee Rotations
3. Waist Rotations
4. Hip Rotations
5. Torso/Arm Swings
6. Overhead Swings
7. Arm Stretches
8. Neck Stretches
9. Arm Circles/Chops
10. Lift the Sky
11. Straight Leg Kicks
12. Heel Kicks
13. Toe Kicks
14. Chin to Toe
15. Tiger Crouches Downward (low single whip)

TAI CHI CHUAN STANDARD STANCES

1. OPENING: Feet are shoulder width apart, parallel to one another with toes pointing forward.

2. INSIDE EMPTY: With flexed knees, one foot is placed lightly along side the other which is supported by the opposite leg.

3. TAI CHI STANCE: Place the heel of the non-weight bearing foot forward in line with heel of supporting foot. The supporting knee is flexed.

4. BOW AND ARROW: Moving from the Tai Chi Stance slowly, shift the weight from the rear to the front leg. Both feet will be flat on the ground, with toes pointing forward and back toes at a 45 degree angle. Heels will be in line with each other, knees flexed, and hips forward. Body weight is distributed with 80 % front and 20 % back.

5. ROLL BACK TO THE TAI CHI STANCE: Moving from the Bow and Arrow Stance, shift 100% of the weight to the rear leg and place the heel of the non-weight bearing foot in line with the heel of the rear leg.

6. HIGH LOTUS: Moving from the Tai Chi Stance, turn the front toes away from the body between 45 and 90 degrees depending upon your flexibility, with the front knee flexed. Shift 90 % your weight to your front leg, leaving 10 % on the

toes of your rear foot.

7. HOOK STEP: Moving from the Tai Chi Stance, turn your front toes inward toward your body and turn 180 degrees, shifting your weight onto the rear foot and into the Tai Chi Stance.

8. SINGLE WHIP: Step into an Inside Empty Stance with the left foot and extend the right arm side-ways to the right at shoulder level. Form a Hook with the right fingers. The left arm is bent with the palm facing upward at the right shoulder.

9. Step with left foot (West) into a Tai Chi Stance and slowly shift your weight into the Bow and Arrow Stance as the left elbow moves left extending towards the left at a 45 degree angle. The left palm faces rotates outward as it moves left until it is fully extended to 180 degrees.

10. GOLDEN ROOSTER: The forearm raises upward with fingertips pointing upward, raise the right knee with foot handing naturally, as if connected by a string. The supporting leg is straight. Repeat on both sides.

TAI CHI STANDARD WALKING STEP

1. Bow and Arrow Stance
2. Roll Back into Tai Chi
3. Step into High Lotus Stance adjusting from 45 degree to 90 degree able.
4. Take a Tai Chi Step
5. Roll forward into a Bow and Arrow
6. Turn the rear toes in to 45 degrees.

Repeat the 6 steps in succession for several practices. Move slowly and fluidly, with flexed knees and good posture maintaining a center of gravity.

TAI CHI STANDARD HAND POSITIONS

1. OPEN PALM: The hands are relaxed yet slightly curved with a space between the fingers and in line with your wrist.

2. FIST: Close fingers lightly so that your thumb folds over your second and third fingers and are in line with your wrist.

3. Hook or Monkey Paw: Crook your hand inward with all 5 fingers gathered together at the tips and slightly rounded.

The Master knows the secret of how to persevere, yet how not to exhaust himself

the I Ching

THE TWENTY FOUR STEP SEQUENCE OF THE PEKING STANDARD YANG STYLE SHORT FORM

Opening

Wild Horse Separating/Combing the Mane
Wild Horse Separating/Combing the Mane
Wild Horse Separating/Combing the Mane

White Crane Flapping/Spreading It's Wings

Brush the Knee, Twist the Waist and Push, left
Brush the Knee, Twist the Waist and Push, right
Brush the Knee, Twist the Waist and Push, left

Playing the Pipa

Stepping Back, Repulse the Monkey, right
Stepping Back, Repulse the Monkey, left
Stepping Back, Repulsing the Monkey, right
Stepping Back, Repulsing the Monkey, left

Grasp the Bird's Tail, left
    1. Ward Off
    2. Pull Back
    3. Press
    4. Push
Grasp the Bird's Tail, right
    1. Ward Off
    2. Pull Back
    3. Press
    4. Push

Simple Cloud Hands
Single Whip
Complex Cloud Hands, Single Whip
High Pat on Horse
Heel Kick, right
Double Temple Strike
Heel Kick, left
Low Single Whip, left
Golden Rooster Standing on One Leg, right
Low Single Whip, right
Golden Rooster Standing on One leg, leg
Fair Lady Weaving/Works at Shuttle, left
Fair Lady Weaving/Works at Shuttle, right
Needle as Sea Bottom
Fan Arm
Turn Around, Parry, Block, and Punch
Apparent Closing/Close Like Shut
Closing

Standard Tai Chi Yang Style 24 Step Peking Yang Form

As taught by Master Richard Kosch

Opening Wu Ji Posture (North)

Feet shoulder width apart.

1. Arms rise up slowly to shoulder height.

2. Forefinger and thumb form triangle; triangle pulls in toward chest and hands push down to Tan Tien, as knees bend, slightly. (It is important to try to keep this height during the entire practice of the form).

Transition (North)

1. Shift weight to RF; step LF to an inside empty stance; simultaneously as if to "hold a beach ball on the right side of the body, with the RH on top, left hand on bottom as if holding a ball.

Separating/Combing the Wild Horse's Mane (West)

1. Step left heel into a Tai Chi stance (West); align heels. Take a half-step.

2. Shift weight into Bow & Arrow (80/20) as RH arcs forward and pulls back; LH arcs upward to block face, Combing the Wild Horse's Mane. (Face West)

3. Turn back toes inward; align heels.

4. From the Bow & Arrow, roll back to a Tai Chi stance.

5. Turn LF 90% (or 45 % for knee problems); form a beach ball on left (LH on top). Take care to maintain balance. Maintain flexed knee position.

6. Step right heel into Tai Chi stance (West).

7. Shift weight slowly into Bow & Arrow stance (80/20) as LH arcs forward and pulls back ; RH arcs upward to block face, Combing the Wild Horse's Mane.

8. Turn back toes in; align heels.

9. From Bow & Arrow, roll back to Tai Chi stance.

10. Turn RF 90%; form beach ball on right with RH on top.

11. Step left heel into Tai Chi stance (west).

12. Shift weight slowly into Bow & Arrow, (80/20) as RH arcs forward and pulls back; LH arcs upward to block face, Coming the Wild Horses Mane.

13. Turn back toes in; align heels.

White Crane Spreading Its Wings (West)

1.Take half step up with RF. Shift weight forward

2. RH (palm up), thrusts under left elbow (bend at the elbows) as left palm pulls in and pushes down between right arm and chest; arms separate; right palm turns outward and stretches upward (above the right temple); LH stretches downward and stops above the left thigh (fingers point inward).

3. Shift weight to RF with LF in an outside empty stance (West).

Brush the Knee, Twist the Waist and Push (West)

1. Thumbs turn away from body. Palms turn up at shoulder height.

2. Right palm drops down to right thigh and continues to circle in back up to shoulder height as the left palm pushes up, blocks back and stops at the right shoulder, palm facing back. The torso and head follow movements to the right.

3. LF takes a Tai Chi step; right arm bends at elbow; (take a half-step); LH drops down to the right side of the waist.

4. Proceed to shift LF slowly into Bow & Arrow; bush the knee with LH, twist the waist, push right palm forward.

5. Turn back toes in; align heels. Face West.

_____

1. From Bow & Arrow, roll back to Tai Chi stance.

2. Shift LF 90 degree into High Lotus stance.

3. Left palm drops down to left thigh and continues to circle in back up to shoulder height as right palm pushes up, blocks face and stops at left shoulder, palm facing back with torso and head following movements to the right.

4. RF takes Tai Chi step; left arms bends at elbow; RH drrops down to left side of waist.

5. Proceed to shift RF slowly into Bow & Arrow; Brush the Knee with RH, twist the waist, push left palm forward.

6. Turn back toes in; align heels. Face West.

———————————

1. From Bow & Arrow, roll back to Tai Chi stance.

2. Shift RF 90 degrees into High Lotus stance.

3. Right palm drops down to right thigh and continues to circle in back up to shoulder height as left palm pushes up blocks face and stops at right shoulder, palm facing back with torso and head following movements to R.

4. LF takes Tai Chi step; right arm bends at elbow; LH drops down to right side of waist.

5. Proceed to shift LF slowly into Bow & Arrow; Brush the Knee with LH, twist the waist, push right palm forward.

6. Turn back toes in; align heels. Face West.

———————————

Playing the Pipa (West)

1. Take a full step up with RF. (right toes next to LF)

2. RH makes a small outward circle to right side ("wax on"); LH pushes back making larger circle to the left side ("wax off").

3. With arms in a 180 degree position, begin to pull right palm into left inside elbow; shift weight to RF as left heel steps into Tai Chi stance. Face West.

Transition (West)

1. Lower left toes down into a flat footed empty stance. (no weight on the LF).

2. Pull right forearm to right waist (palm up) and push LH forward blocking the face. (Face West).

Step Back Repulse the Monkey (West)

Step Backward East

1. Right palm flips behind at shoulder level.

2. Bend right arms at elbow; turn left palm upward, and step back with left toe.

3. Shift weight to LF as RH pushes forward and left, slowly, forearm pulls to waist height, (turn waist R to L)

Front toe forward; align heels. (Face West)

Next portion:

1. Left palm flips behind at shoulder level.

2. Bend left arm at elbow; turn right palm upward, and step straight back with right toe, slowly.

3. Shift weight to RF as LH pushes forward and right forearm pulls to waist level. (turn waist L to R) Front toe forward; align heels. (Face West)

Continuing:

1. Right palm flips behind at should level.

2. Bend right arm at elbow; turn left palm upward, and step straight back with left toe, slowly.

3. Shift weight to LF as RH pushes forward and left forearm pulls to waist level. (turn waist R to L)
Front toe forward; align heels. (face West)

Last portion:

1. Left palm flips behind at should level. 2. Bend left arm at elbow; turn right palm upward, and step straight back, slowly with right toe.

3. Shift weight to RF as LH pushes forward and right forearm pulls to waist level. (turn waist L to R)
Front toe forward; align heels. (face West)

*Please note that there are 4 repetitions to the "Step Back Repulse the Monkey" sequence.

Transition (North)

1. Right palm flips behind at shoulder level.

2. Step LF to inside empty stance.

3.Bend right arm at elbow to form beach ball position on right (RH on top).

Grasping the Bird's Tail (West)

1. Step to a Tai Chi inside empty stance. Take a half step, roll forward, hands move as the body rolls forward to Ward Off.

2. LH rises, RH lightly touches L wrist to follow Left elbow, bent at 45 degree. Palm is towards face.

3. Palms turn over. Hands pull back to the Right hip. (Shift weight back into a Tai Chi Stance with LF)

Transition to Press:

Right palm up, reaches backwards at shoulder height. LH rotates so that thumbs are pointed 90 degrees upward.

Rear, (right) hand moves forward to re-enforce left wrist with base of fingers to Press. Fingers point upwards.

1. Take 1/2 step forward to a Bow and Arrow Stance, to Press. (LF forward)

2. Hands separate, palms forward, drop palms down to waist level.

3. Roll back to a Tai Chi Stance with LF. Thumbs and Index fingers form a triangle with the hands moving upward to "Call" with elbows up and outward.

4. Tuck elbows inwards, take a 1/2 step to roll forward to "Push" with elbows down.
Transition: RH reaches back, turn left toes in, shift to Left Foot Inside Empty Stance.

Hold the Beach ball with RH on bottom, LH on top.

Grasping the Bird's Tail (East)

1. Step to a Tai Chi inside empty stance. Take a half step, roll forward, hands move as the body rolls forward to Ward Off.

2. RH rises, LH lightly touches R wrist to follow Right elbow, bent at 45 degree. Palm is towards face.

3. Palms turn over. Hands pull back to the Left hip. (Shift weight back into a Tai Chi Stance with RF)

Transition to Press:

Left palm up, reaches backwards at shoulder height. RH rotates so that thumbs are pointed 90 degrees upward.

Rear, (left) hand moves forward to re-enforce Right wrist with base of fingers to Press. Fingers point upwards.

1. Take 1/2 step forward to a Bow and Arrow Stance, to Press. (RF foreword)

2. Hands separate, palms forward, drop palms down to waist level.

3. Roll back to a Tai Chi Stance with RF. Thumbs and Index fingers form a triangle with the hands moving upward to "Call" with elbows up and outward.
4. Tuck elbows inwards, take a 1/2 step to roll forward to "Push" with elbows down.
Transition:

LH reaches back, turn Right toes in, shift to Right Foot Inside Empty Stance.
Hold the Beach ball with LH on bottom, RH on top.

Sifu Rich's Notes:

The 5 arm movements; Ward Off, Press, Pull Back, Call and Push are all wonderful segments to practice individually in order to improve balance during weight transfers.

Transition (North)

1. Pull left heel in toward body; right palm faces down at Tan Tien; Left palm faces downward at chest level,
fingers pointing inward toward body, but they don't overlap.

Simple Cloud Hands (North)

1. Shift weight to LF as arms shift left, palms down, turning right toes inward. (hips remain facing North)

2. At full extension, ((RH under L elbow), change palm height; face left palm down at Tan Tien, (turn the waist) palms facing downwards at chest level. Do not overlap hand movements.

3. Shift arms to right side as weight shifts to right.

4. RH with Right arm fully extended forms a Hook. Left palm is up at the R shoulder.

5. With full weight on RF, step LF into an Inside Empty.

Single Whip (West)

1. Step Left heel into Tai chi Stance, (align heels). (West).

2. Shift weight into Bow & Arrow; left elbow (45 degree angle)

3. Take 1/2 step, turn back toes in; align heels.

Transition (North)

1. Pull right heel inward; RH hook opens.

2. Slowly shift weight to the Right foot; turn Left toes inward (North). Left palm drops downward to Tan Tien and continues upward to front of Right shoulder, palm facing chest; Right palm down at Tan Tien. (don't overlap movements of hands).

Complex Cloud Hands (North)

1. Shift arms Left as weight shifts to LF. At full extension, palms turn over; change palm height; turn waist and step to RF Inside Empty Stance.

2. Shift arms right as weight shifts to RF with LF Inside Empty.

3. At full extension, palms turn over; change palm height, turn waist as LF steps Left. (Left palm faces chest; Right palm faces down at Tan Tien. Hand movements should not overlap. Shift arms left as weight shifts to LF.

4. At full extension, palms turn over, change height and step to Right Inside Empty Stance. (Right palm faces chest; Left palm face down at Tan Tien. Don't overlap the hand movements). Shift arms right as weight shifts to RF with LF Inside Empty Stance.

5. At full extension, RH makes a hook; LH comes to the Right shoulder, palm up.

Single Whip (West)

1. Step L heel into a Tai Chi Stance. (align heels) (West)

2. Take 1/2 step, shift weight into a Bow & Arrow Stance; Left elbow (45 degree angle) leads the way as Left palm extends left (West)

3. Turn back toes in: align heels

High pat On Horse (West)

1. Take 1/2 step up with RF as RH hook opens

2. Turn both palms upward as you look at the RH.

3. Right arm bends at elbow as L palm pulls inward at waist level and R palm pushes forward (West).

4. Shift weight back to RF with LF into an Outside Empty

Heel Kick (South) (Kick to Right)

1. Back of LH thrusts across back of Right wrist.

2. With LF, shift weight into High Lotus (face South)

3. Left palm turns outward; arms separate outward and down to Tan Tien.

4. Continue to circle arms upward; left right knee comes up; kick to the Right (West)

5. As right heel kicks (West), arms chop downward (180 degrees).

Double Temple Strike (West)

1. LH circles overhead to meet RH (face West).

2. Take Tai Chi step with RF (face West)

3. As arms drop down to waist level, turn palms upward; at thigh level, make fists; shift to Bow and Arrow; circle arms outward; Double Temple Strike with fists.

Heel Kick (South) (Kick to Left)

1. As fists open, shift weight to LF: turn Right toes inward (South), as LH circles overhead; arms 180 degrees.

2. Circle arms downward as LF steps to inside empty.

3. As arms circle upward, lift left knee up and kick to the Left.

4. As Left heel kicks (East), arms chop downward (180 degrees).

5. Hook RH as LH arcs over to Right shoulder (left palm facing West) and swing Left leg into Golden Rooster.

Low Single Whip (South)

1. As LF steps left, sink downward on Right leg. With RH hooked, turn Left palm

toward face and drop LH downward over extended Left leg.

2. Turn Left toes forward (East); shift weight to Left leg and drag RF into Bow and Arrow Stance.

3. Turn Left toes outward 45 degrees; Left palm down: RH opens.

Golden Rooster Standing On One Leg (East)

1. Pull LH back to waist (palm down) as Right elbow pulls Right knee up. Standing on Left leg (RH fingers pointing upward).

Transition (North)

1. Drop right toe to outside empty; pivot on ball of LF.

2. LH hooks; RH comes to Left shoulder (palm faces West).

Low Single Whip (North)

1. As RF steps right, sink downward on Left leg. With LH hooked, turn Right palm toward face and drop RH downward over extended Right leg.

2. Turn Right toes forward (East); shift weight to Right leg; drag LF into Bow and Arrow.

3. Turn right toes outward 45 degrees; Left palm down; LH opens.

Golden Rooster Standing on One Leg (East)

1. Pull RH back to waist (palm down) as left elbow pulls left knee up. Standing on Right leg. (Left fingers pointing upwards).

Fair Lady Weaving at Shuttle (East)

1. Step Left hell into a Tai Chi Stance. Take 1/2 step

2. Turn LF to High Lotus and form beach ball (LH on top)

3. RF steps into Tai Chi Stance; take a 1/2 step and shift slowly into Bow and Arrow Stance as LH blocks upward in front of body and stops at temple as RH pushes forward (East).

Needle at Sea Bottom (East)

1. Take a full step up with RF, toes near Left heel.

2. Extend Right fingertips forward (thumb up), placing Left palm at inside of Right elbow.

3. Right arm drops to the right side as LH clears off, down.

4. As the body turns slightly to Right, make a small circle in front of the body with LH; Follow movement of RH as it circles back and overhead; bend right wrist, elbow, and continue to thrust fingers downward to floor, with left palm at Right, inside elbow, Left fingers upward.

5. Shift weight to RF; LF (toes) to outside empty.

Fan Arm (East)

1. Turn Right palm upward and lift arms to shoulder height; Left palm at Right inside elbow.

2. Step Left heel into Tai Chi Stance.

3. Turn Right palm away from body (thumb down).

4. Take 1/2 step and roll forward into a Bow and Arrow as RH pulls back to temple and LH pushes forward (align heels) (East).

Turn Around, Parry, block and Punch (West)

1. Fist RH; shift weight to right leg as right arm opens (arms 180 degrees). Turn Left toes in (face South).

2. Shift weight back onto LF as RF steps to Inside Empty Stance. (Face South).

3. LH blocks upward at left temple as RH (fist eye up) circles down and then up to Left side of waist.

4. LH clears down across body, past right elbow and fist.

5. RF takes a Tai Chi step (West). Right fist arcs over Right leg; continue RF to High Lotus, bringing fist to Right side of waist, blocking with LH in front of body, palm facing North.

6. LF takes Tai Chi step (West)

7. Roll forward to Bow and Arrow and Punch. (RH is fisted with Left palm at inside of Right wrist).

Apparently Closing (West)

1. Place LH under Right fist; open RH

2. Shift weight back to RF dragging LF back into a Tai Chi Stance as palms turn outward and draw back to "Call".

3. LF takes 1/2 step; roll into a Bow and Arrow and "Push" hands forward (West)

Closing (North)

1. RH arcs overhead as weight shifts to RF. Turhn left toes inward (North).

2. Shift weight to LF as both hands circle downward.

3. RF steps shoulder width apart as both hands cross at Tan Tien, LH on top.

4. As arms circle upward to head level, slowly straighten legs; palms turn downward; forefingers and thumbs form a triangle.

5. Hands push down to Tan Tien and separate.

6. Stand quietly for several moments.

Thank you for your continued practice of

Tai Chi Chuan

Ultimate Grand Fist

Master Richard Kosch
10th Degree

Master Rich's Reading Suggestions:

Anything by Grandmaster T. T. Liang

The Tai Chi Boxing Chronicles by Kuo Lien Yang

T'ai chi Ch'uan by Da Liu

(Da Liu is credited as being the first to bring Tai Chi to the US in the 1950's).

Master Kosch is also the author of Tai Chi Principles for Massage Therapy.

May Your Tai Chi Journey Be Long.........